FAST FACTS SERIES

What to Do When You Have Type 2 Diabetes

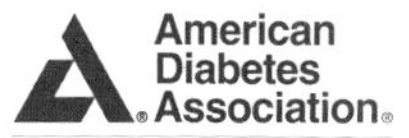

Director, Book Publishing, John Fedor; *Editor,* Laurie Guffey; *Production Manager,* Peggy M. Rote; *Composition*, Circle Graphics, Inc.; *Cover,* Design Literate, Inc.; *Printer,* Port City Press.

Printed in the United States of America
1 3 5 7 9 10 8 6 4 2

Consult a health care professional before trying any of the suggestions in this publication. ADA assumes no responsibility for any injury that may result from the suggestions or information in this publication. To purchase this book for special sales, write:

Lee Romano Sequeira
American Diabetes Association
1701 North Beauregard Street
Alexandria, Virginia 22311

Contents

This Can't Be True!

"No way!" "Not me!" Your feelings about having diabetes are completely normal. You're not alone. More than 16 million people in the U.S. have diabetes, and 5 million of those have it but don't know it.

Actually, it's a good thing you were diagnosed.

There are important things for you to start doing right now to prevent complications down the road. The more you do to stay healthy—eat right, be more active, take diabetes pills or insulin (if you need them), and quit smoking—the better you'll feel, and the less diabetes will bother you. It's up to you. What you do every day really matters.

So What Is Diabetes?

If you know what it is, it's easier to understand what you need to do. Your body turns the food you eat into glucose (sugar) to use for energy. The glucose goes into your bloodstream to travel around to all the body cells. But, if you have diabetes, the glucose can't get into your cells. It has to stay in your blood, causing "high blood sugar."

You may have been feeling tired, sluggish, breathless, or very thirsty. Other symptoms are:

- dry, itchy skin
- frequent urination
- blurry vision
- sores that don't heal well
- numbness or tingling in fingers or toes
- problems with sexual function

What Is Insulin, Then?

Insulin is made by your pancreas, and its job is to help glucose get into your body cells. If you have diabetes, either you aren't making enough insulin, or the insulin you have isn't working very well. This is called insulin resistance, and can happen if you are overweight. If you're overweight, you may have too much body fat for the amount of insulin you make. This is why losing weight makes high blood sugar disappear. Even with a 10-pound weight loss, the insulin works better. But your high blood sugar will be back if you gain weight again.

Is There a Difference between Type 1 and Type 2 Diabetes?

People with type 1 diabetes don't make any insulin and must take insulin every day to survive.

People with type 2 diabetes do make some insulin but it doesn't work well. Some people with type 2 take extra insulin. Some take pills, and some control diabetes by eating the right foods and exercising.

Why'd I Get It?

Maybe diabetes runs in your family. Maybe you are overweight or never exercise. Maybe you're American Indian, African American, or Latino. Maybe you're older than 45, or had gestational diabetes when you were pregnant.

All these put you at risk, but no one really knows why you have it and your neighbor doesn't. If you know someone else at risk, tell him that healthy eating and exercise can **prevent** diabetes, too!

The Right Tools For the Job

The best tools for managing your diabetes are:

- a healthy meal plan
- an interesting exercise program
- diabetes pills or insulin, if you need them
- records of blood sugars, food, and exercise
- helpful health care providers
- ways to reduce stress

You can still eat your favorite foods. You have to move some more. You have to check your blood sugar levels, learn what to do if they are high or low, and see your doctors regularly.

If you do these things, you'll be delighted with how good you feel—better than you've felt in years. Just try one small change you can stick to . . . and then one more and then one more, until you're where you want to be!

But What Can I Eat?

First, take a deep breath . . . no need to panic. You can eat a great variety of foods. You can still eat your favorite foods—in moderation. You can still have a glass of wine or beer. You can still have dessert. Feel better?

What's the Plan?

You need a plan—a meal plan. You design one with a registered dietitian (RD). You need to do this right away. A good meal plan that you like (and will use) is your key to success. By the way, if your life has a big change (for example, you get pregnant or retire), then your meal plan needs to change, too. Go see an RD and be honest about your likes and dislikes. He or she can get you started on the right path.

A diabetes meal plan is no different from any other healthy meal plan—same foods, same quantities. The problem is that many people in this country have terrible eating habits. We eat way too much, period, but especially too much fat and too much fast food.

Poor eating is just a habit. It's a shortcut . . . but it won't take you where you want to go. Get a meal plan based on:

- what you like to eat and drink
- your daily schedule, including work and exercise
- what you weigh now and what you want to weigh

A healthy meal plan includes all food groups: grains, fruits, vegetables, meats, meat substitutes, and dairy products. Here are three ways to create a meal plan—the pyramid, exchanges, and carb counting.

The pyramid scheme. No, it's not really a scheme. It's a way to picture what foods you should eat and how much of them to eat. Food is divided into 6 groups and put into the sections of a pyramid, called the Food Guide Pyramid. The American Diabetes Association developed the one on page 8 just for you. You eat more of the foods in the wide base and fewer servings of the foods in the smaller sections at the top.

The healthy base of the pyramid is grains, beans, and starchy vegetables. Eat 6 or more servings of these each day. You get 5 servings in all from the fruit (2 servings) and vegetable (3 servings) sections of the pyramid. Moving up to the narrower sections, you get a little meat and milk, 2–3 servings of each. (Thomas Jefferson said he liked just enough meat to be a condiment to his vegetables. Try thinking about meat that way.) Finally, eat only a small amount of fats, sweets, and/or alcohol each day. This may turn out to be more food than you're used to eating—especially if you skip breakfast or lunch—but spread over 3 meals and a snack, it's a healthy way to eat.

The exchange system. There are 7 different exchange lists of foods: starches, fruit, milk, other carbohydrates, vegetables, meat, and fat. All the foods on a list have the same amount of carbohydrate, protein, fat, and calories. The math is done for you, so you can "exchange" or trade one food for another in your daily meals.

Your meal plan tells you the number of exchanges to eat at each meal and snack. For

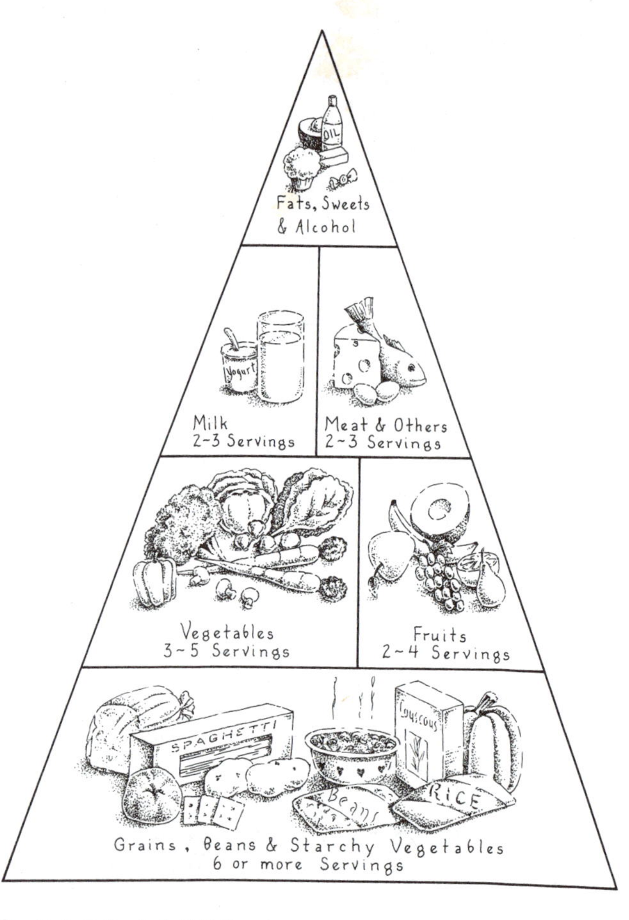
OIL
Fats, Sweets
& Alcohol
Yogurt
Milk
2-3 Servings
Meat & Others
2~3 Servings
Vegetables
3~5 Servings
Fruits
2~4 Servings
SPAGHETTI
Couscous
Beans
RICE
Grains, Beans & Starchy Vegetables
6 or more Servings

example, breakfast might be 2 starches, 1 fruit, and 1 milk. You choose foods you want from the exchange lists to make up your meal.

Count 'em. No, not calories. Count grams of carbohydrate. It is the carbohydrate in food that raises your blood sugar. Desserts, popcorn, potatoes, bread, rice, fruits, milk, and vegetables all contain carbohydrate (carb).

Oops! You've probably heard that people with diabetes can't eat sugar. We used to think that a sweet dessert would make blood sugar go much higher than a baked potato. Now we know that the **same amount** of carbohydrate—no matter what food it comes from—makes your blood sugar go up about the same.

There are no forbidden foods, and dessert can be part of your meal plan. You don't have to feel deprived or different, but you do have to make wise food choices—more vegetables than dessert, more fresh foods than processed ones. Why? Because whole grains and vegetables give you the vitamins, minerals, and fiber you need. They're premium fuel for your body.

How do you count carb? First, find out how many grams (g) of carb are in the foods you eat.

- Each starch, fruit, and milk exchange has 15 g carb. A vegetable serving has about 5 g carb (another reason to eat more veggies).
- Nutrition Facts on a food label tell you grams of carb as Total Carbohydrate. (Ignore the grams of sugar—they're part of the Total Carb.)
- BONUS: If you eat 5 or more grams of dietary fiber (part of Total Carb), subtract that number from your carb grams for the meal. (This is another benefit of high-fiber foods such as whole grains, fruits, and vegetables!) Fiber slows down the rise in blood sugar.
- Double-check the serving size. If you're actually eating two servings, you're getting twice as much carb as is on the label.
- For the thousands of foods without a label, buy (or check out the library) books listing carb and fat gram counts. Newer cookbooks have this information, too.

Nutrition Facts

Serving Size 1 cup (228g)
Servings Per Container 2

Amount Per Serving

Calories 260 Calories from Fat 120

	% Daily Value*
Total Fat 13g	**20%**
Saturated Fat 5g	**25%**
Cholesterol 30mg	**10%**
Sodium 660mg	**28%**
Total Carbohydrate 31g	**10%**
Dietary Fiber 0g	**0%**
Sugars 5g	
Protein 5g	

Vitamin A 4% • Vitamin C 2%

Calcium 15% • Iron 4%

* Percent Daily Values are based on a 2,000 calorie diet. Your daily values may be higher or lower depending on your calorie needs:

	Calories:	2,000	2,500
Total Fat	Less than	65g	80g
Sat Fat	Less than	20g	25g
Cholesterol	Less than	300mg	300mg
Sodium	Less than	2,400mg	2,400mg
Total Carbohydrate		300g	375g
Dietary Fiber		25g	30g

Calories per gram:
Fat 9 • Carbohydrate 4 • Protein 4

Next, find out how much carb to eat. For most adults, it's 4–5 carb servings at each meal, or 60–75 g carb in each meal (1 serving = 15 g carb).

It's better to eat your daily carb spread over three meals than to eat it all at dinner and send your blood sugar sky high.

Actually, try to eat the same amount of carb at the same meal each day. Your blood sugar should fall into a pretty predictable pattern.

You Mean I Can't Just Ignore That Thing?

The Nutrition Facts label gives you valuable information about serving size, calories, fat, carb, and sodium. Some labels even give food exchanges. Use these labels when you're choosing foods.

I can only have HOW much?

MEASURE your serving sizes. Most of us eat two and three times as much as we think we're eating. The only way to be sure is to measure it.

Here are some "hand-y" ways to see servings:

- A meat serving = the palm of your hand.
- A tablespoon = the tip of your thumb.
- One cup = your fist.

Actually, if you eat one cup of rice, you're eating 3 servings. One serving is 1/3 cup. You're eating 45 g carb. Larger servings mean more carb, which can surprise you with high blood sugar.

For 1 week, weigh or measure all you eat. Then you'll be able to eye your plate and judge the correct serving sizes. Once a month, weigh and measure to be sure your servings are not creeping up.

Tips to reduce servings

- Don't put serving bowls on the table.
- Use smaller plates and bowls.
- Use the right size glass for the job (4-oz juice glasses rather than 12-oz tumblers, for example).
- Drink liquids with your meal to feel full.

- Chew each bite slowly, 20 times. It takes 20 minutes to feel full.

I Don't Know How to Cook Like This!

Yes, you do. You just didn't have a good enough reason to try healthy tips before now.

First, reduce the fat

- Use low-fat salad dressings, cheeses, milk, and sour cream. (Watch for the extra carb in low-fat products.)
- Solid margarine has unhealthy "trans" fats, which are bad for your heart. Try a bit of butter or oil.
- Use nonstick cookware.
- Cook food in 1 Tbsp or less of olive or canola oil.
- Use nonstick cooking spray, wine, or low-fat or fat-free broth instead of oil.
- Buy lean cuts of meat. Trim visible fat before cooking. Avoid eating poultry skin.
- Roast, grill, or broil meat on a rack.

Check your favorite recipes. Experiment to see how the flavor changes when you use less fat. Use yogurt or fruit purees to give texture to baked goods. Use fat-free evaporated milk to make things rich and creamy. Try recipes from diabetes cookbooks and use those same techniques and ingredients in your favorite recipes. If the carb count is too high, eat a smaller serving. A smaller piece of your favorite pie may satisfy you more than a large piece of the low-fat version.

The Doctor Says I Have to Lose Weight

You will. If you see a dietitian, get a realistic meal plan, and use it, you will lose weight. Move around more, too. There's nothing magical about successful weight loss. You have all the tools you need right now.

Losing weight is one of the best things you can do. Losing weight helps your body use insulin better, so your diabetes control improves. It brings down high blood pressure without medication and lowers your risk of heart disease. If you lose enough weight, you may even be able to cut back on your insulin or diabetes pills. Hooray!

But how do I do it? Get a meal plan and an exercise plan. Together they are the perfect weight loss plan.

- Shoot for losing only 1–2 pounds a week.
- Celebrate each goal achieved–with a movie, a new book, a pair of earrings, golf?
- Waste NO time on regret if you slip. Get back on your meal plan at the next meal.
- Keep a food diary for a week. Write down everything you eat, what time it is, and how you're feeling. See what may be affecting you and adjust your meal plan to fit better.
- Plan for challenges, such as parties or times when you're bored or depressed.
- Find ways other than eating to work out stress.

Do I Really Have to Exercise?

Yes, but exercise isn't sweating or pain or expensive gyms. Exercise is walking up the stairs instead of taking the elevator. It's taking the dog around the block twice instead of once. (Boy, is your dog going to be happy that you were diagnosed with diabetes.) It's seeing your friends on the tennis court, golf course, or at the pool instead of in restaurants. Run the vacuum, wash the car, garden for an hour. It all adds up to exercise.

Exercise is the magic "pill" everyone is looking for. Exercise lowers your blood sugar levels naturally, so you may not need as much insulin or pills. Exercise lowers your blood pressure, reduces stress, and cuts your risk of heart disease. Exercise is the triple whammy you can use on diabetes.

Well, That Sounds Okay . . . How Do I Start?

By seeing your doctor . . . to find out if there's anything you shouldn't do. Once you get the go-ahead, start small and build up slowly. Start with something you like. If you can't decide, start walking (see chart on p. 19).

To walk, you need only shoes that fit well. Or try swimming, biking, or low-impact aerobics. And don't forget dancing, playing football with your grandchildren, and yoga.

If you have pain in your calves while walking, rest and then walk some more. Exercise improves your circulation, so this pain—which is caused by poor circulation—will gradually go away.

Exercise enough to make your heart beat a little faster. Don't fall down in exhaustion or be in such discomfort that you avoid ever exercising again, but move so you feel an increase in your heart rate. Be able to carry on a conversation while you exercise.

Stop if you are dizzy, short of breath, sick to your stomach, or in pain. Maybe you're going too fast or need a drink of water or some carbohydrate. If you're going to tune up your body, you have to learn to listen to it.

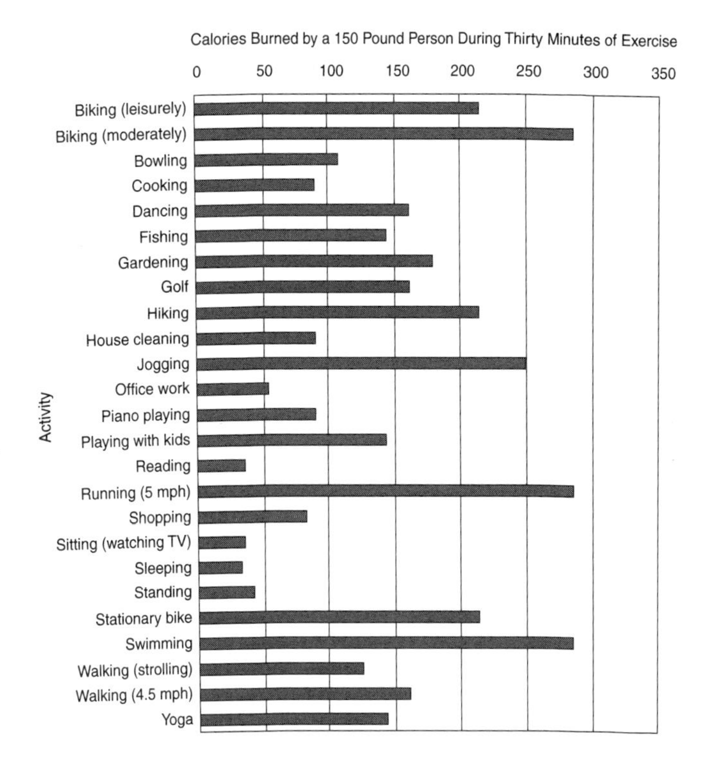
Calories Burned by a 150 Pound Person During Thirty Minutes of Exercise
0
50
100
150
200
250
300
350
Activity
Biking (leisurely)
Biking (moderately)
Bowling
Cooking
Dancing
Fishing
Gardening
Golf
Hiking
House cleaning
Jogging
Office work
Piano playing
Playing with kids
Reading
Running (5 mph)
Shopping
Sitting (watching TV)
Sleeping
Standing
Stationary bike
Swimming
Walking (strolling)
Walking (4.5 mph)
Yoga

But What Kind of Exercise Should I Do?

The three types of exercise work together:

- aerobic (such as jogging)
- strength (such as lifting weights)
- flexibility (such as stretching)

Aerobic exercises use your heart, lungs, arms, and legs. They reduce body fat and help you lose weight.

Strength exercises make your muscles stronger and your bones sturdier, so you're less likely to become injured. BONUS: Muscle burns calories and lowers your blood sugar even when you're resting. You want more muscles!

Flexibility exercises keep your muscles and joints limber, so you can keep moving like a youngster.

Learn the right way to do exercises you choose. Learn how to use any equipment. Wear safety gear, such as goggles or a helmet.

If you are a real beginner, start with a 1-minute walk every day. Listen to your body. Add 1–5 minutes to your walks each week. Slowly build up to 30 minutes a day, 3–4 days a week. You can break it up into three 10-minute walks or six 5-minute walks. It all counts. (A pedometer is a fun tool that counts how many steps you take each day! 2,000 = 1 mile.)

Best Foot Forward

Wear clean cushioned socks made of "wicking" fibers. No wrinkles. Choose shoes designed for the exercise you plan. Check your shoes before you put them on for nails or rips in the lining. After exercising, check your feet for blisters or cuts. If you have nerve damage, you may not feel an injury to your foot. So you have to look and touch to feel it.

Look for redness. Redness may mean your shoes rub or are too tight or there is a thick seam in your sock. Call your doctor if you have any foot problems.

When to Check Your Blood Sugar

Exercise makes blood sugar go down naturally.

If you take insulin or certain diabetes pills (sulfonylureas and meglitinides), exercise can make your blood sugar level go too low. Check your blood sugar before and after exercising. Always carry a carb-containing drink or glucose tablets with you to treat low blood sugar!

When you'll be exercising 30 minutes or more, check blood sugar before you begin. If your blood sugar is low, you may need a 15-g carb snack. If it's high, drink extra water to flush out the sugar. Check your blood sugar if you feel weak or shaky or if you've been exercising for more than 1 hour.

Your blood sugar can fall for 10–24 hours after exercising. Keep an eye on it, especially during the night or the next day.

You may need 1/2 cup of milk, juice, or a sports drink; a piece of fruit; or cheese and crackers if you exercise more than 30 minutes at a time. After exercise, you may need a snack. Talk with your health care team about what to eat for snacks and when to eat them.

If you take insulin, you can also lower the dose on the days you exercise. Ask your health care team for help with this.

Drink water before and after exercise—and during strenuous exercise—to avoid getting dehydrated. You can go farther and longer if you have plenty of water to drink.

You MUST carry identification that clearly states you have diabetes. Carry drinks or food for low blood sugar plus instructions for other people on how to treat your low blood sugar.

You could find yourself in a life-threatening situation if the people around you don't know what to do to help you. Tell your aerobics instructor or exercise buddies how to help if you can't do it for yourself (page 44).

How to Stick With It

You'll find it easier to stick to your exercise program if you make exercise as regular as sleeping and eating. Find a buddy to go to class with you or walk with you at lunchtime. Making the commitment to meet someone for exercise can help get you out the door.

Choose an exercise workout that you can do with little travel time and preparation. Find things that fit easily into your daily routine. (They add up!) (See chart on page 25.)

In the beginning, select an activity that doesn't require special equipment, clothes, or fees. Check on exercise classes at community rec centers, churches, and schools, where prices are usually lower.

Set goals you can measure. Instead of saying your goal is to "begin exercising," give more details. Say "I'll walk for 15 minutes on Monday, Wednesday, and Friday after lunch." Gradually increase your exercise times. If you're bored, try something new!

ACTIVITIES FOR THE NONEXERCISER

When you are on your feet and moving around, you are using 2 to 3 times more energy than when you are sitting. Here are some ways to get moving:

- Get up to change TV channels instead of using the remote.
- Do the ironing while watching TV.
- Walk around your house during TV commercials.
- Wash dishes, load the dishwasher, or load the clothes washer or dryer during commercials.
- Sweep your sidewalk.
- Use a rake rather than a leaf blower.
- Use a shovel instead of a snow blower.
- Use a push lawn mower rather than an electric one.
- Plant and maintain an herb or vegetable garden.
- Take your pet for a walk.
- Play actively with children.
- Volunteer to work for a school or hospital.
- Walk to the subway or bus stop.
- Take the stairs rather than the elevator.
- Stand or walk around while you're on the phone.
- Walk during lunch, during your break, while the oven is preheating, or while waiting for your prescription.
- Run errands that require walking, such as grocery shopping.
- Park your car farther away from your destination.
- Take a walk with someone you want to talk to.

What's This Pill For?

If you're depressed about needing to take diabetes medication, try looking at it this way. Almost everybody has to take some kind of medication. If your medication (along with healthy eating and exercise) keeps your blood sugar under control, you'll be healthier for many years. That's great!

Keeping your blood sugar levels under control helps your heart, eyes, feet, and kidneys stay in good working order.

Why Do I Need Drugs?

Some people with diabetes don't make enough insulin and need a pill to help them make more. Some make enough insulin but their bodies are resistant to it. They need a drug that makes their cells more sensitive to insulin (and more open to glucose). Some people have both problems.

How many are there? Drugs have a scientific name, a generic name, and a brand name. The table on page 28 shows the names of different drugs for diabetes.

How do they work? Drugs work in different ways. The table on page 31 shows how the different diabetes drugs work in the body.

Alpha-glucosidase inhibitors, biguanides, and the 'glitazones help insulin work better, so your body gets more out of the little it makes. These drugs should be taken with meals. For example, **acarbose** and **miglitol** delay absorption from your intestines of the carb you've eaten, which lowers your blood sugar after meals. Besides getting glucose from the food you eat, your body makes glucose in the liver. **Metformin** causes the liver to make less glucose, which lowers your blood sugar. And **pioglitazone** and **rosiglitazone** make your muscle cells take up more insulin, which lowers blood sugar, too.

Sulfonylureas and **meglitinides** increase your supply of insulin, which lowers your blood sugar. They can cause it to go too low, so you'll need to check your blood glucose more often and **always** carry a snack with you (page 43).

MEDICATIONS AVAILABLE TO TREAT DIABETES

Alpha-glucosidase Inhibitors	Acarbose Miglitol	Precose Glyset
Biguanides	Metformin	Glucophage
Meglitinides	Nateglinide Repaglinide	Prandin Starlix
Sulfonylureas	Glimepiride	Amaryl
	Glipizide	Glucotrol
	Glyburide	DiaBeta Glynase Micronase
	Tolbutamide	Orinase
	Tolazamide	Tolinase
	Chlorpropamide	Diabinese
'Glitazones	Pioglitazone Rosiglitazone	Actos Avandia

Watch Out for Side Effects

Some drugs cause allergic reactions. Any type of skin rash—redness, itching, swelling, or hives—that develops after you start a new drug could mean you are allergic to it. This is especially true of **sulfonylureas**. Call your doctor right away if you suspect you are allergic to a drug.

Common side effects of **acarbose** and **miglitol** are flatulence, stomachache, and diarrhea. If you take a lower dose, symptoms may go away. If you take **metformin**, you may not feel hungry or feel nauseated, or have diarrhea. Some people on **pioglitazone** and **rosiglitazone** retain fluid and gain weight. Tell your doctor right away if you have any side effects. Be aware that any diabetes drug can make you gain weight because your blood sugar control improves, and you stop losing glucose (calories) in your urine.

Watch Out for Drug Interactions

Yes, the drugs you take for diabetes can interfere with drugs you take for other conditions, or vice versa. For example, at high doses, aspirin can increase the effectiveness of **sulfonylureas** and surprise you with low blood sugar.

If you're taking **sulfonylureas**, you may not be able to drink alcohol. Within 10–30 minutes of drinking alcohol or taking a medicine that contains alcohol, you may get a headache, flushing or tingling in your face, nausea, or light-headedness.

Tell your doctor if you want to have alcohol occasionally while on **sulfonylureas**. Your doctor may be able to prescribe a different drug or tell you why you need this one.

Anytime your blood sugar goes out of control for no apparent reason and you have recently changed your medication, think about a drug interaction. But don't stop taking a prescription drug until you've talked to your doctor.

Carry all your pill bottles in a bag to your doctor's appointment, so your health care team can see every drug you're taking. Try to go to the same pharmacy, so there is an accurate record of everything you're taking. Then the pharmacist's computer should warn him or her of any possible drug interactions.

HOW DIFFERENT DIABETES MEDICATIONS WORK

Medication Class	Site of Action	Action
Alpha-glucosidase Inhibitors (e.g., Acarbose or Miglitol)	Digestive system	Slows the breakdown of starches to glucose. Slows the entry of glucose into the bloodstream after a meal.
Biguanides (e.g., Metformin)	Liver	Decreases glucose production by the liver.
Meglitinides (e.g., Repaglinide)	Pancreas	Stimulates insulin release by the pancreas in response to a meal.
Sulfonylureas (e.g., Glyburide or Glipizide)	Pancreas	Stimulates insulin release by the pancreas.
'Glitazones (e.g., Pioglitazone or Rosiglitazone)	Muscle	Enhances glucose uptake by the muscle.

What If Pills Don't Work?

Your doctor may prescribe a diabetes pill or two different pills. You may start on a low dose and go higher or start high and then lower your dose. Some drugs take many weeks before they start working. Ask if yours is one of these.

If one drug doesn't lower your blood sugar well enough, another might. Or your doctor may prescribe a combination of insulin and diabetes pills. Diabetes pills generally work best for people who have had type 2 for less than 10 years.

Diabetes pills cannot take the place of your meal and exercise plans. In fact, if you don't eat healthy and exercise, too, diabetes pills may not work for you.

If your doctor has tried every pill and combination of pills but your blood sugar is still too high, don't worry. You can take insulin to get better control of your diabetes and avoid diabetes complications.

I Don't Want to Go on Insulin!

You may not have to, but about 40% of people with type 2 end up going on insulin. Most people hate the idea of insulin for two reasons: they think their diabetes must be much worse, and they're afraid of having to give themselves a shot.

Well, your diabetes is not necessarily worse if you have to take insulin. Sometimes pills just stop working. Don't blame yourself, and don't feel guilty. We don't know why a pancreas wears out. Going on insulin is just another treatment . . . and it's very effective—which means better health for you. Don't put it off!

As for the needles . . . have you seen them? They're TEENSY. They're also lubricated, so when you learn to inject properly, it is pretty painless.

There are "injection aids" on the market if you are squeamish about the needle itself. You hold one of these devices against your skin, and it inserts the needle for you. There are insulin "pens" where you can dial in the dose you want and tiny needles deliver it. There are insulin pumps that automatically deliver insulin through a tiny tube. And soon—perhaps very soon—you'll be able to *inhale* insulin.

Types of Insulin

Insulin types are grouped by their time of action, which has 3 parts: onset, peak, and duration.

- Onset is how long insulin takes to start working.
- Peak time is when insulin is working hardest.
- Duration is how long insulin keeps working.

Most insulin is called human insulin and is grown in a lab. There are four types of insulin to copy how the body produces insulin in spikes at meals and in tiny amounts over the day and night.

- **Rapid-acting** insulin (lispro or insulin aspart) starts working in 5 minutes. It works hardest in about 1 hour and stays in the blood 3–5 hours. This is like the insulin your body naturally produces in response to food.
- **Regular insulin** starts working 30 minutes after you take it. It works hardest 2–3 hours after you take it, and stays in your blood 4–6 hours.
- **Intermediate-acting** insulin (NPH or lente) takes 2–4 hours to start. It works hardest from 4–12 hours after your shot, and lasts 14–20 hours.
- **Long-acting insulin** (ultralente or glargine) starts working 6–10 hours after you take it. It stays in your blood for 20–24 hours.

Each person responds differently to insulin. The action times may be different for you. Your doctor will help you develop an insulin plan that matches your meal and exercise plan.

It's important to eat and exercise on schedule when you're on insulin. If you take your bedtime insulin but skip your snack, for example, your blood sugar may go too low during the night.

If you exercise especially hard but don't lower your insulin dose or eat more carb, your blood sugar will go too low.

On the other hand, if you eat a bigger meal than usual, you may not have enough insulin to cover the food and your blood sugar will be high.

You can buy different combinations of insulin or mix them yourself. For example, at breakfast, you might mix rapid-acting insulin to cover the meal with intermediate-acting insulin to last all day.

Insulin Storage and Safety

You need to store your insulin in the refrigerator. You have to protect it from extreme heat or cold and from getting knocked around. Check the expiration date before opening your insulin. You don't want to take something that has lost its effectiveness, or you'll get high blood sugar.

Look at the insulin in the vial before you use it. If it's regular insulin, it should be clear, with no floating pieces or color. NPH, lente, and ultralente are cloudy, but with no floating pieces or crystals.

Traveling with Insulin

If you're traveling by car, pack a cooler with ice, snacks, and insulin. (Be sure the insulin doesn't touch the ice or freeze.)

Pack a diabetes supply bag that includes:

- a letter from your doctor stating that you have diabetes
- copies of all your prescriptions
- your diabetes pills
- insulin, syringes, and your injection supplies (For air travel, insulin must be in the original box with the prescription label on it.)
- snacks for 24–48 hours (close at hand)
- blood sugar meter and strips
- glucagon kit (for low blood glucose emergencies)

If you're flying and crossing time zones, going east gives you a shorter day. You may need less insulin. Westward travel gives you a longer day. You may need more insulin. Your health care team can help you plan how to adjust insulin for this.

Remember to wear your medical ID when traveling and always carry food with you. Be prepared and you won't be upset by delayed or cancelled meals.

I Can't Remember All This!

Yes, you can. Work closely with your health care team. They will help you learn how to mix and give yourself insulin. They can help you with the bigger challenge of learning to balance insulin with food and exercise. (Insulin and exercise lower blood sugar. Food raises it.) If you check your blood sugar level and keep good records, you have the information you need to select foods, the insulin dose, and when and how long to exercise, so you can avoid wide swings in your blood sugar.

Some Days I'm Low, Some Days I'm High

The best way to keep track of how well your diabetes is doing is to check your blood sugar. Instead of simply saying "I feel fine" or "I feel lousy," you can check it, record it, and use your records to fine-tune your diabetes care.

Checking helps you find out what happens to your blood sugar when you eat certain foods (such as pizza or pecan pie), when you exercise, or when you lose or gain weight. It helps you see what happens to blood sugar when you take diabetes pills or insulin, are sick, or are emotionally upset.

A blood check can help you decide whether to eat a snack, take more insulin, or to exercise.

Some people do not feel any symptoms when their blood sugar goes too high or too low. Checking helps them know what's going on. If you keep careful records of your blood sugar checks, you and your health care team have an easier time figuring out which diabetes pills or insulin work best for you.

How to Check

Check your blood sugar with a glucose meter. Blood sugar is measured in mg/dl. (Mg/dl means milligrams of sugar per deciliter of blood, which is like saying teaspoons of sugar in a gallon of blood.)

Your doctor will help you choose your own blood sugar goals. Target ranges are often 80–120 mg/dl before meals and 100–140 mg/dl before bedtime, but you may need higher ranges to avoid going too low.

You use a lancet to get a tiny drop of blood from the side of your finger, forearm, or thigh for the test strip or meter. The meter gives your blood sugar number in 15–120 seconds, depending on which meter you use.

With visual strips, you wait, wipe the blood away, and hold the strip next to a color chart. The chart gives a range of blood sugar numbers. Visual strips are only a backup—for example, if the battery in your meter goes dead when you're on a trip.

Follow the instructions for your meter. Ask your health care team to recommend one for you—AND to help you learn to use it.

When to Check

The more you check, the more you'll know about yourself.

- If you treat diabetes with a meal plan and exercise only, you can check before breakfast and, occasionally, 2 hours after a meal to see how high blood sugar rises after you eat and if it returns to normal in the morning.
- If you take diabetes pills, check before breakfast. If you check twice a day, vary the time of the second check.
- If you take insulin, check 2–4 times a day. Check before breakfast and vary the other checks, but one should be 2 hours after a meal.

A urine test cannot take the place of blood checks because it can only show that your blood sugar was high hours ago. Blood checks show what your blood sugar is right now.

Keep Records

To fine-tune your diabetes care, you need a week of records with the results of glucose checks, date, and time. Write them even if your meter has a memory. Also record the foods you eat, when you eat, and when you exercise.

If the glucose number was high or low, write what was special about that day. Did you change your meal plan? Did you skip an insulin injection or forget to take your pill? Were you under a lot of stress or unusually active?

Work with your doctor or educator. Do your results seem too high or too low for no reason? Do you need to calibrate your meter? Is it time to change your meal plan, or exercise, or medication?

When to Call the Doctor

Call the doctor if:

- your blood sugar stays above 250 mg/dl (or the level your doctor gives you) for several hours
- you are unable to follow your meal plan for more than 24 hours
- you can't get low blood sugar to go away

Low Blood Sugar

The scientific name for low blood sugar is hypoglycemia. You can have this problem only if you take insulin or certain diabetes pills (sulfonylureas or meglitinides). You may feel strange or pass out. Your warning signs may be different from someone else's. If you feel any warning signs, eat 15 grams of carb and then check your blood sugar to see if it is too low.

Excellent foods to treat hypoglycemia are:

- 1/2 cup fruit juice or regular soft drink (not diet)

- 4 teaspoons granulated sugar
- 2 tablespoons raisins
- 1 tablespoon honey or syrup
- 2–3 glucose tablets
- 1/2 tube glucose gel or cake frosting

After treating your low blood sugar with a snack, wait 15 minutes and check your blood sugar again. If it's still low, eat another snack.

If it is more than 1 hour before your next meal, have a glass of milk or half of a meat sandwich after you treat your low blood sugar.

Treating Severe Lows

If you take diabetes medicines that can make your blood sugar too low and you don't treat it, you might pass out. Teach your co-workers, family members, and friends to give you a carb drink or snack, even if you act angry or stubborn.

If you are not awake or can't swallow, you need a shot of glucagon. Glucagon is a hormone that raises blood glucose. It has to be injected. Your doctor can prescribe a glucagon kit for you.

You will need to train your co-workers, family members, and friends to give you the shot.

To avoid THAT drastic situation, check your blood sugar often, and treat lows right away! Things that can cause low blood sugar are:

- skipping a meal or snack
- not eating all of your meal or snack

LOW BLOOD GLUCOSE WARNING SIGNS

- Anger
- Anxiety
- Blurred vision
- Clamminess
- Clumsiness
- Confusion
- Fatigue
- Headache
- Hunger
- Impatience
- Irritability
- Light-headedness
- Nausea
- Nervousness
- Numbness
- Pallor
- Pounding heart
- Sadness
- Shakiness
- Sleepiness
- Stubbornness
- Sweating
- Tension
- Weakness

- not eating at the right time
- exercising harder than usual
- drinking too much alcohol
- taking too much insulin

Find out what causes *your* blood sugar to sink and find ways to avoid it. It may take a few unpleasant experiences before you learn to juggle things better to prevent low blood sugar.

High Blood Sugar

The scientific name for this is hyperglycemia. You can go for years without knowing your blood sugar is too high. But high blood sugar levels do damage to your body over time—endangering your eyes, heart, kidneys, feet, circulation, and nerves.

High blood sugar can happen if

- you eat too much
- are sick or under stress
- do not exercise
- do not take your insulin or diabetes pills

High blood sugar levels make you thirsty and you urinate more, as your body tries to get rid of the sugar. Be sure to drink plenty of water when your blood sugar is high.

If your blood sugar is more than 240 mg/dl for more than 24 hours, call your doctor. If your level is above 500 mg/dl, go to the hospital immediately.

When you're ill, you don't eat and exercise as usual. These changes—plus the stress of the illness itself—can cause high blood sugar. Work out with your doctor what you should do.

Drink plenty of fluids. It is important not to get dehydrated. Check your blood sugar more often until it is under control.

But I'm Gonna Try (And Here's Why)

Were you struck with fear when the doctor told you about your diabetes? Did you think of stories you've heard about people losing their feet? Going blind? Damaging their kidneys?

Those stories come from the time before we knew how to control blood sugar. Now we know how to prevent, slow down, and treat diabetes complications. Complications are caused by high blood sugar over a long time. **If you control your blood sugar levels** with a plan (eating right, exercising, taking diabetes medication, not smoking, and defusing stress), **you have the strongest chance of preventing or postponing (or reversing) the complications of diabetes.**

You may not want to read about diabetes complications. But you need to learn how to take care of yourself now, so you don't have to worry about what's down the road.

An Ounce of Prevention

Get these regular checkups:

- Yearly dilated eye exam for retinopathy
- Yearly urine test for protein
- Every 6 months, feet examination (your provider will check for loss of feeling, change in shape, or poor circulation)
- Yearly blood test for cholesterol and other fats

The best way to prevent problems (besides keeping your blood sugar under control) is to get regular checkups. Then you'll find any problems early. This means you'll get early treatment, which increases your chances of healing and success.

Most people with type 2 diabetes have 2 regular checkups a year. Your doctor will order a blood test called an A1C test. This test shows your average blood sugar level over the past 2–3 months. (You can't change the results by fasting before the test.) The chart on the next page tells you how often to see your doctor and which tests you need.

Sometimes, you may see other diabetes specialists: a nurse or diabetes educator to learn how to check your blood sugar or give insulin, a dietitian, an eye doctor (ophthalmologist), a foot

RECOMMENDED FREQUENCY OF MEDICAL EXAMS AND TESTS

	Every 3 Months	Every 6 Months	Every Year	Every 2–3 Years	As Needed
Regular Visits* If not meeting goals	●				
If meeting goals		●			
Physical Exam			●		
Dilated Eye Exam			●		
Lipid Profile (Blood fats test) If last reading was abnormal			●		
If last reading was normal				●	

A1C Test If not meeting goals or if treatment changes	●				
If meeting goals		●			
Kidney Tests			●		
Urine Tests			●		
Thyroid Tests					●
Electrocardiogram					●

*Regular visits include measurement of your height, weight, and blood pressure, a foot exam, an eye exam, and a check on anything that was abnormal at a previous visit.

doctor (podiatrist), an exercise specialist, and a psychologist.

Eyes. The back of your eye, or retina, is like the film in a camera. Years of high blood sugar levels can harm the retina, causing retinopathy. At first, diabetes weakens the blood vessels in the retina, but vision is not hurt at this stage.

Sometimes, blood vessels start to leak. Fragile new vessels grow, but in the wrong places or leak, too. Your vision may not change, so you don't know there is a problem. That's why it's important to have regular dilated-eye exams. If retinopathy is found early and treated with laser surgery, it is tamed. If eye problems are not treated, they can lead to loss of vision.

What you can do for your eyes

- Keep blood sugar and blood pressure under control.
- When you are diagnosed with diabetes, get a dilated-eye exam with drops in your eyes to make the retina easier to see.
- Get follow-up exams your doctor advises.

- If your doctor finds eye disease, see an ophthalmologist familiar with diabetes-caused retinopathy right away.
- Laser surgery is quick, nearly painless, and very effective.

Kidneys. The blood in your body passes through filters in the kidneys to remove waste materials. Wastes go into the urine.

Your kidneys can be hurt by the extra sugar in your blood that goes through them over the years. Some people with diabetes are prone to kidney disease. High blood pressure can also make kidney disease worse.

What you can do for your kidneys

- Keep your blood sugar under control.
- Keep your blood pressure under control. (Try for 130/80.) Stop smoking. Cut salt in your food. Exercise. Don't drink alcohol. Take blood pressure medication.
- Have a yearly test for protein in your urine once a year. This test is for "albumin."

- Get other kidney tests your doctor recommends. These might be for "creatinine," "urea nitrogen," or "BUN."

Nerves. Nerves carry messages from one part of your body to other parts. They tell your body what you see or feel. If you touch something hot or step on something sharp, nerves let you know.

High blood sugar can damage nerves. Parts of your body, such as feet or genitals, may not feel as well as they once did. Or nerves can send phony pain signals.

Nerve problems can cause diarrhea, urinary tract infections, sweating (especially after eating), dry skin, light-headedness, or loss of balance. If you have any of these problems, talk with your doctor.

What you can do for your nerves

- Keep your blood sugar in control. Getting better control can reverse some of the nerve damage.

- Look at and touch your feet every day. If your nerves are not working as they should, you can injure your feet and not know it.
- Avoid drinking too much alcohol.

Heart and blood vessels. Problems with your heart are MUCH more common in people with diabetes. That's because the sugar in your blood makes it sticky. And sticky blood can lead to heart attack, stroke, or poor blood flow in your arms and legs. Circulation problems can make it more difficult for men to have erections.

But don't despair—there are things you can do right now to keep your heart and circulatory system healthy.

What you can do for your heart and blood vessels

- Keep your blood sugar in control.
- Keep your blood pressure under control. (Try for 130/80.) Cut salt in your food. Don't drink alcohol. Take blood pressure medication.
- Exercise.

- Keep your blood cholesterol under control. If it is higher than 200 mg/dl, consider medication.
- Follow a healthy meal plan low in saturated fat. Try olive oil and nuts as your fat choices per day.
- If you're overweight, lose some!
- Exercise (with your doctor's guidance).
- If you smoke, STOP IT.

Feet. Diabetes can harm nerves in your feet. You may not feel a cut or injury to your foot. Or your feet might hurt even when there is no injury.

Diabetes can also slow down the flow of blood to your feet. Your feet may get cold, blue, or puffy. Cuts on your foot may take longer to heal.

Foot problems are serious. Don't try to treat them yourself. See your doctor.

What you can do for your feet

- Check your feet every day for redness, sores, or swelling.
- Keep your blood sugar under control.

- Call your doctor if you have pain in your feet; a cut that won't heal; dry, cracked skin; or unexplained high blood sugar that could be caused by an infection in your foot.
- Wash your feet every day and dry well, especially between your toes.
- Wear shoes that fit well. Try running shoes.
- Cut your nails around the shape of the toe. File edges gently.
- If you can't see or can't reach your feet, have a podiatrist take care of them.
- Use lotion on dry areas (not between your toes).
- Check the inside of your shoes before you put them on for rips, tacks, or stones.
- Don't soak your feet, go barefoot, wear tight socks or shoes, break blisters, use hot water bottles or heating pads, or remove corns yourself.

A Balancing Act

Since controlling blood sugar is so important to prevent complications, you need to know what makes your blood sugar go up or down.

- **Food** makes blood sugar go up. Following your meal plan keeps it from going too high or staying up too long.
- **Diabetes pills or insulin** make blood sugar go down.
- **Exercise** makes blood sugar go down. Your blood sugar goes down while you exercise and for up to 24 hours afterward.
- **Stress.** Being worried, excited, or angry can make blood sugar go up. A stress on your body, such as being tired or sick, can also make blood sugar go up.

Picture a scale with food and stress on one side, and insulin, pills, and exercise on the other. When your diabetes is in good control, the scale is balanced. But any change can tip the scales. An extra snack or a fight with someone can drive blood sugar up. Too much insulin or more exercise than usual can lower your blood sugar too much.

Do what you can to keep your scale in balance. Follow your meal and exercise plan and take the right amount of diabetes pills or insulin on time. Do you know some good ways to reduce stress?

You might try a few of these:

- Find someone to talk to. Join a support group.
- Take a walk or play a sport (exercise!).
- Join a book or movie group.
- Take up a hobby or volunteer to help others.
- Get away for a night or weekend.
- Soak in a warm bath or read a good book.
- Listen to some great music.
- Dance.
- Learn to say no.
- Practice breathing deeply.
- Get a massage.
- Rent a funny movie.
- Eat wisely.
- Sleep on it.

About the American Diabetes Association

The American Diabetes Association is the nation's leading voluntary health organization supporting diabetes research, information, and advocacy. Its mission is to prevent and cure diabetes and to improve the lives of all people affected by diabetes. The American Diabetes Association is the leading publisher of comprehensive diabetes information. Its huge library of practical and authoritative books for people with diabetes covers cooking and nutrition, fitness, weight control, medications, complications, emotional issues, and general self-care.

To order American Diabetes Association books:
Call 1-800-232-6733. http://store.diabetes.org
[Note: there is no need to use www when typing this particular Web address]

For more information about diabetes or ADA programs and services:
Call 1-800-342-2383.
E-mail: Customerservice@diabetes.org